GET DESIRED TRAITS IN FETUS

A BOOK FOR EVERY PREGNANT WOMAN

SHAILA RAO

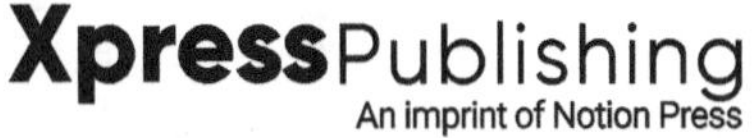

XpressPublishing
An imprint of Notion Press

Old No. 38, New No. 6
McNichols Road, Chetpet
Chennai - 600 031

First Published by Notion Press 2019
Copyright © Shaila Rao 2019
All Rights Reserved.

ISBN 978-1-64678-117-1

Contents

Disclaimer

My self Shaila Rao

Declare that what ever counseling for pregnant women I am doing is on the basis of my experience on myself and by counseling other pregnant women. Also on the basis of experience shared by other mothers in my survey.

What ever scientific basis I have given is possiblity. It is by reading general magazines,results of research work found in news papers.etc.

There is no such guarantee for any favourable or unfavourable results on fetus.

As such I am not answerable to any judiciary matter.

There are lot many other things effect the fetus.

CHAPTER ONE

INTRODUCTION

I am a free lancer. I worked after consulting Doctors and psychologists.

Myself Shaila Rao .

B.Sc.(science biology) , M.A in Psychology.

From Indore (M.P).

India.

Hypothesis

" Effect of deliberate

thinking and keeping in mind traits by pregnant women, on fetus. "

I have prepared a card for pregnant women, it is a sort of ala- carte , for pregnant women. I am attaching that too with this.

I have attached scientific basis also with diagram.

According to my study, pregnant women, like in computer can programme whole life of fetus from birth till death.

The traits thought during pregnancy occur in the life of fetus one after another.

Brief account of my research study is thus

1) My work is 43 years old. Started working on this in 1976 March.

2) It is research based.

3) It has got scientific and genetic basis.

4) I experimented on myself twice. With the aim to tell the world if I am benifited.

5) My research study was presented in National mental health conference in 2008, in Indore. Sponserd by UGC govt of India.

6) Before starting counselling to other pregnant women, I surveyed 120 mothers of different age group and socio economic status.

7) Then after getting published in local news papers and tv channel, I started counselling other pregnant women and doing follow up study. I am

counseling pregnant women since 1992.

8) Till now I have counselled around 200 pregnant women.

9) This counselling can be carried on with the help of different media. ie print media, audio visual media, internet etc.In print media I have got album and card to help pregnant women to get better results for baby in fetus.

Example of my counselling: -

A pregnant woman has to think and keep in mind all good positive traits in mind.

1)She has to think that my baby should be smiling ,cheerful, active.

2) My baby should be intelligent.

3) My baby should do its home work and preparation of tests, exams etc on its own.

And many many more traits.

Like this the traits may or may not be genetic. Still they occur. The genetic explaination is there.

My main aim to reach maximum pregnant women and help them to get good child. Let us build a better generation and help the human kind to make an ideal world.

A pregnant woman can not only get the desired traits in fetus, but also she can decide i.q level, quantity of food child will have, physical features and physique, can decide career for fetus, avoid diseases, can control daily routine physiological habits like digestion, excretory system, sleep system etc etc.

Advantages.

 Now pregnant women can get desired traits in fetus

We can get better generation

We can build an ideal world.

Will be of great benefit to individual, society ,and mankind.

Introduction of my topic

Effect of deliberate Thinking and keeping traits in mind during Pregnancy

From many hundreds of years the effect of thinking during pregnancy been a very important feature. Even from the time of super power lord Krishna   (from Abhimanyu's birth and pregnancy of his mother - Subhadra when he was in womb and learning the tactics of War in the womb.

Imagine if she had listened how to defend and come out, whole Mahabharat would have changed.

Leaving aside this to be a Mythological concept, but now with scientific basis, it can be said that if pregnant Woman thinks deliberately or keeps in mind positive personality trait both physical and psychological in mind that occurs in baby in fetus.At the same time she can avoid negative traits also.

By accepting this phenomena pregnant woman can be happy, can lead better kind of life for child also, it will be better to have good qualities from the time of birth. Ultimately this may help to build an ideal world.

In this phenomena pregnant woman can select the qualities, better to select from – herself, husband, grand parents of the baby in fetus. (Considering the genetic factor)

CHAPTER TWO

NORMS OF THINKING

Every body's mind is like an ocean, same is the mind of pregnant woman. Many thoughts are coming and going. Till now it was going on randomly. Now I have tried to give a structured thinking to pregnant women. I have given some norms of thinking. I want it should be called "SHAILA'S NORMS" of thinking for pregnant women.

I counsel age wise of baby.Here pregnant woman can programme whole life of fetus. It will be shown by fetus,when it comes in this world time to time.

1. **When the Child is born:** When the baby is born how it should be – it should be cheerful, active, smiling, good looking, healthy (resistance to cough, cold, indigestion i.e. should digest properly) Should be chubby. Should be always smiling. Should sleep well at night. Keep itself clean. Should have good sharp eye movement.should be very intelligent.

2. **When the child is around six months :** Three months onward child should posses good responding system. Should look here and there. Should be very active. Around six months should develop good grasping power. Should be sharp, intelligent.

3. Around Two and half years should have liking to go to school, if admitted should go to school nicely, happily.

a. In school should pay attention to teachers, whatever is teacher teaching should have concentration. Should concentrate on what teacher is teaching, even at home while studying should concentrate on studies only. Should retain in mind whatever has been taught. Even revise after returning to home. Express nicely whatever has been taught orals and in written when taught, when grow up. In written, expression should be there understand the question and should answer to the point and whatever required.

b. Should do its Home work on its own

c. Should prepare and learn all the things for test and exams quite in advance by itself.

d. Should keep all the books and note books properly in place and bag neatly. Should take care of study materials nicely.

e. In higher classes should have planning how to study what to study etc. On the whole should be very intelligent like father or mother   (whoever is more intelligent) or anybody else like close relative. Should be very sharp in answering, Should be bold in viva and interviews. Should like to answer in class.

Should be career conscious. Should read study material books, join classes related to its career. Should have knowledge of current affairs, G.K etc. Should be hard working in studies.

4. **Extra Curricular Activities :**Besides studies in school, should be or not should be interested in other activities like Sports, Debate, Quiz, Puzzles, Speech, Music, Dance, Painting or time being Monitor or head Monitor etc. It is up to pregnant woman to select any one of them. Relatively other qualities/ traits should occur like talk debate. Should be bold stage. Should prepare debate material from books. For sports should be strong enough and

Some pregnant woman feel, extracurricular activities should not be so much involved, because it will be hectic for child and studies will be at less.

5. **Favorite Pass Time**: When the baby gets some   time how it should pass it. For example reading books, playing a while, painting, Social work, Evening walk, Gardening, Watching T.V. talking to somebody with family members or neighbors. It can be like this when child should play a little with friend in the evening when grown up anything from above,

6. **Eating Habits:**Should eat all nutritious things. Should have liking for milk, salad, Green vegetables etc. Vegetarian or non-vegetarian according to pregnant wish.

    While eating should concentrate on eating. Should eat average neatly and cleanly. When goes to other caste or other people, place   according to them. Should be ready for simple meals like – khichadi, Sandwich only rice and dal. Should be a little self dependent in cooking so that when mother or wife or cook is away need not stay hungry.

7. **Dressing Up Habit**: Should have good dressing up habit according to time and fashion. Should dress up neatly and cleanly.

    Should keep ones own cloth neatly in wardrobe or Almirah. Even should look after washing, ironing of clothes. While going out of station should manage ones own packing.

8. **Money Spending Habit:**Pregnant woman should keep in mind regarding money spending habit, should be such that average money spender. Should have habit of saving a part of earnings. Should save properly like in bank or recurring deposit. But should love to spend on close relative and fast friends and on self.

9. **Making Friends:**Baby when grows up should like to make friendship with people having good habits, good nature. Should sometime keep friendship or mixed up with people of all ages. Fast friendship with one or two. Give and take relationship with few but hi and bye with others.

10. **In problematic situation:** Should handle the situation intelligently and carefully with calmand peacefulmind. Should study the situation and take decision accordingly. If required in hot discussion should be bold and balanced, State of mind and answer or scold in few words, so that the other person keep mum or become speechless.

11. **Inter relationships:**Should love, respect, caring sharing with parents grandparents, brother and sisters. Take care of parents in old age. In marriages and other family functions, should mix up with all relatives.

12. **Physical features and physique and Complexion:** To select physical features like pointed nose, big eyes, husband's/wife's/ grandparent's complexion, thick hair, straight or curly, good teeth alignment, forehead, shape of fingers nails, feet etc. Physiques – nor too fat not too thin, good physique stout, flat tummy, strong and energetic body.

13. Should have good character, should have one life spartner

14. Should be positive thinker

15. **Career**

How to remove negative traits
SHOULD BE,   IS RIGHT.
SHOULD NOT BE,   IS WRONG
To remove negative trait Pregnant woman should honestly analyse self and husband and surrounding, if there is any negative trait should think opposite of it. May be it related to physical features, IQ ,nature , habits ,etc.

Suppose pregnant woman and her husband are dusky. She should think my baby should be fair.

Pregnant woman's mind is simple tool which help her to get desired traits in fetus. Can write fate of the fetus. This tool we can control with our counseling. This counselling is a sort of remote control for her mind.

Beside these above mentioned qualities pregnant woman should keep in mind all other good qualities of herself, husband, parents, inlaws, brother, Sister etc.

इन उपरोक्त गुणों के अलावा गर्भवती महिलाओं ने स्वयं के, पति के, आई बहनों, माता पिता एवं सास - ससुर के सभी सिर्फ अच्छे गुणों को मन में रखना चाहिए।

Pregnant woman should not keep any negative trait in her mind, even if it comes should think opposite of it. Suppose if laziness comes to mind think, baby should be active. If angry think calm and cool headed.

गर्भवती महिलाओं को कोई भी नकारात्मक गुण मन में नहीं रखना चाहिए, अगर कोई नकारात्मक गुण मन में आए तो उसका विपरीत सोचना चाहिए - जैसे आलस का विपरीत - चुस्त, गुस्से का विपरीत शान्त स्वभाव।

Looks & Features — शिक्ल में कैसा हो

My baby should be good looking, Fair Complexion, Sharp Pointed Nose, Lovely Thick Hair, straight or curly, colour of hair can also be selected , Beautiful strong eyes even teeth, always fit health, Height and Average Physique can be thought. (Colour of Eyes, Hair and Dimple on Cheeks or Chin can be thought)

THIS COUNSELLING HAS FOLLOWING FEATURES :

- This counselling is based on experimenting on self (Shaila Rao) in 1976 twice.
- A survey on 120 mothers of different age groups and socio - economic status was done in 1998 while sharing their pregnancy experiences.
- More then 150 pregnant woman have been counselled and follow up study was done. The thought traits were found occurring.
- This counselling has possible Biological / Genetic basis.
- This study was presented in 2008 at the National Mental Health Conference held at Indore.
- This counselling is general sharing of experience, does not have any type of guarantee. It is for the welfare of society and mankind. The Biological basis is collected from ordinary news papers, magazines, books and TV channels etc. Hence not answerable to any court or judiciary.

इस काउंसलिंग से संबंधित जरूरी जानकारियां :

- यह काउंसलिंग स्वयं पर किए गए प्रयोगों पर आधारित है।
- 120 अलग अलग माताओं के अनुभवों पर आधारित है।
- यह काउंसलिंग 150 से अधिक गर्भवती महिलाओं की काउंसलिंग करने के पश्चात्‌ किए गए अनुभवों के आधार पर है।
- इस काउंसलिंग के लिए कुछ वैज्ञानिक आधार सामान्य अखबार, पत्रिकाओं, टीवी चैनलों पर दिए गए प्रसारण पर आधारित है।
- इस काउंसलिंग का उद्देश्य समाज तथा के कल्याण पर आधारित हे तथा किसी भी प्रकार की कानूनी अदालत के लिए जवाबदेही नहीं है।
- यह अध्ययन सन्‌ 2008 में राष्ट्रीय मानसिक स्वास्थ्य सम्मेलन इन्दौर में प्रस्तुत किया गया था।

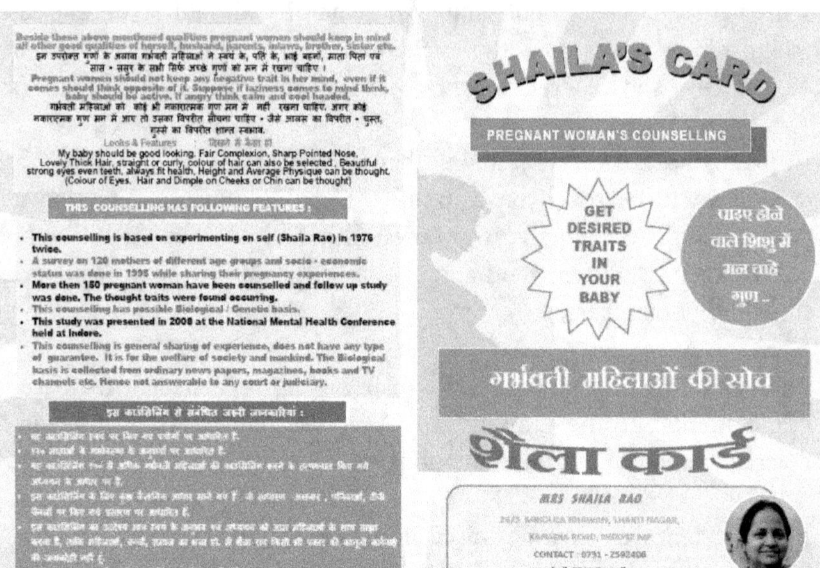

1. My baby in fetus should be smiling, cheerful and active.
मेरा होने वाला शिशु दिखमुख, हमेशा मुस्कुराता, खुशमिजाज और चुस्त हो.

2. When child is school going age he should happily go to school.
मेरा शिशु स्कूल जाने की उम्र में अपने आप राजी - खुशी स्कूल जाए.

3. From the age of 3-4 years my baby should take interest in studies and writing work. Should do its home work, test and exam preparation on its own.
मेरा शिशु चार पांच साल की उम्र से पढ़ाई व सिखने में रूची ले, अपना होमवर्क, टेस्ट व परीक्षा की तैयारी स्वयं करे.

4. My baby should be very sharp and intelligent.
मेरा शिशु बहुत बुद्धिमान और तीव्र बुद्धि का हो.

5. While studying my baby should concentrate on studies.
मेरे शिशु ने पढ़ाई के समय सिर्फ पढ़ाई पर ध्यान दे.

6. Baby should be bold in answering questions and in interviews.
मेरा शिशु क्लास, वाईवा और इन्टरव्यू में हिम्मत और अच्छे से जवाब दे.

7. As my baby grows should be hardworking and devoted towards his studies and work.
जैसे जैसे शिशु बड़ा होता है, पढ़ाई और काम में ज्यादा मेहनती और लगनशील हो.

8. My baby should take good care of study materials.
शिशु पढ़ाई से संबंधित किताबें और अन्य वस्तुओं का अच्छे से ध्यान रखे.

9. At the age of 15 - 16, my baby should be Career conscious.
पन्द्रह सोलह साल की उम्र में मेरे शिशु ने अपने करियर बनाने पर ध्यान देना चाहिए.

10. At the age of 20 - 22 baby should be hardworking and attentive towards making career.
बीस-बाईस की उम्र में पढ़ाई - करियर पर अधिक ध्यान देना चाहिए.

11. My baby should be hard working in job or business.
मेरे शिशु ने नौकरी या व्यवसाय में अच्छा ध्यान देना चाहिए .

12. My baby should be understanding and have feeling of responsibility.
मेरा शिशु समझदार हो और अपनी जिम्मेदारियों को समझना चाहिए.

13. My baby should be calm in problematic situation, should solve the problem boldly and intelligently. मेरा बेबी किसी भी तरह की समस्या आने पर शान्त रहे, समस्या का समाधान हिम्मत और बहादुरी से करे.

14. My baby should be adjustable in all types of circumstances.
मेरा शिशु हर तरह के माहौल में अपने आप को समायोजित करे.

15. In childhood my baby should be little naughty. Should not touch household things.
बचपन में मेरा बेबी थोड़ासा नटखट होता चाहिए पर घर की वस्तुओं को सन्भाल कर चलना है.

16. My baby should use earned money properly and should also save some.
मेरा शिशु कमाए हुए पैसों का सही इस्तेमाल करे, थोड़ी बचत भी करे.

17. My baby should be self dependent, work related to self should do on its own.
मेरा शिशु खुद के काम खुद करे.

18. My baby should be well behaved.
मेरे शिशु ने सब के साथ अच्छा व्यवहार करना चाहिए.

19. My baby should have good grasping power, memory, expressing power and good communication skill. मेरे शिशु में किसी भी बात को अच्छे से समझ कर अच्छी स्मरण शक्ति के साथ दूसरो को अच्छे से बताने की क्षमता होनी चाहिए.

20. In leisure time my baby should read good books, watch TV for little time or any other activity. खाली समय में मेरे शिशु ने अच्छी किताबें, थोड़ी समय टीवी या फिर कोई भी अच्छा कार्य, शाम को टहलने जाना, सामाजिक कार्य आदि करे.

CHAPTER THREE

EXPERIMENTATION ON SELF IST PREGNANCY – 1976

After marriage in 1976 January, I was fresh M.A (psy). When I was pregnant, my relatives told me to read books of great national heroes. One of my close relative said that, your baby will be like father because she had read in Femina that, newly married woman when pregnant is more attracted towards husband and keeps in mind about husband. So this struck to my mind that whatever is in mind that comes in baby. I liked few habits and physique etc. of my husband but few habits I wanted like mine. Then it came to mind, whether the baby is male or female I did not know. So I decided to think of such habits nature and traits which are suitable for both male or female.

I thought my baby should have smiling face, cheerful, active, sharp when born. (It was all exactly same). From six months around should learn, grasping and responding to whatever much more as mentioned in norms and thinking.

Around two and half years should have liking to go to school in that age. All traits I thought that should pay attention, concentration, , grasp retain (come home) say what happened whole day in school. Should do its learning of lessons question answer home work, prepare for test and examination of its own. Should have feeling of responsibility towards studies. I observed above mentioned traits right from the class one. Should be bold enough to stand up and answer to the question asked in the class. (This we both were lacking.)

I had thought the baby should take part in debate, quiz, speech competition etc. My son from the class IV took part in such type of competition till last when he was in M.M.S (Master of Management Science) final year. Took part in all India competition related to management topic at Bombay and stood 1st. left behind IIM Bangalore, Delhi etc. Always throughout his school and college life he took part. We both lacked this traits. In 10thClass he took part in science congress and stood 1stin District.

I had thought that, around the age of 15-16 should be career conscious. Exactly around this age, the trait occurred. I had in mind that to make career should read magazine related to career. He used to read Business Today, India Today etc.

During pregnancy I wanted my child should like maths and do well in maths. Though we both are Bio-students. He disliked Biology and took maths, Science as major subjects. He always scored good and higher percentage in Maths. Also as a time pass he used to do Maths. (Non- genetic trait). Regarding his favorite pass time I had thought reading books, that too good books related to career. Even now he is continuing with the same habit.

I had also in mind that in the evening 2-3 hours should spend here and there with friends. Exactly same habit is there. When young (around 8 years) he used to play a while and he himself used to return home. After growing up also same habit. Whatever making friends – I wanted my child should have friendship with person who like to study, have good manners and good habits. Besides the criteria of rich or poor. Considering friendship with other sex should have healthy friendship no nonsense type running after girls. Should not hesitate to talk to opposite sex.

Eating Habits: Regarding eating habits, my Husband and in-laws side eat non veg. I wanted child too eat Non-veg. He is fond of Non-veg. I liked and wanted child should eat pure ghee. He likes and eats. I had purposely thought, should dislike potato, because my mother in law used to use Potato with every veg and non veg.

Dressing Up habits: My husband has very good style and liking for dresses. I thought it is wastage to purchase too many clothes. I myself is not so much fond of clothes. I wanted, he should have dressing up habit like me. He is exactly the same. He purchases very less clothes that too how much is required.

Money Spending Habit: I wanted he should be like me. First save a little then spend and not extravagant like my husband. This has come true. He saves from his Salary.

The problematic situation: I had thought should be calm and handle the situation intelligently, he is exactly the same. Should never back answer to parents. If parents get angry should explain calmly. (All this traits has occurred).

Inter relationship: I wanted should be caring and respect to parents. My husband was same for his father. I wanted the same to with my husband. He never answers back.

Regarding psychological traits– should be bold in interviews, on stage etc. but decent at home, tolerance like my mother, adjusting type every where, in all situation ambitious all these traits has occurred.

Regarding physical traits: I wanted physique should be like my husband. Hair (straight) like mine, Eyes like mine. Heights at least like my husband

Career : Career wise I had thought child should go for MBA in marketing and get high post at very young age. Same occurred.

CHAPTER FOUR

THOUGHT PROCESS DURING II PREGNANCY

During 2ndPregnancy I had thought few negative qualities. This time I had not thought any thing like smiling face. Rather I had thought should be serious (like my husband). If a girl should be little coward or shy type introvert. But when grown up around 15-16 years, should be bold enough to solve her own problems. One contradictory thing I thought i.e. on one side I thought introvert type but take part in debate etc. This thing has happened , she is introvert, less talking but not only takes part in debate but also has won the laurels. (Prizes, Certificates) she spoke in front of 200 people.

As mentioned above contradictory habit – taking part in debate, occurred.

Regarding study habit – I had thought should learn while playing. When she was in K.G.I from that time, she become teacher and thus learnt all the things. Same as first time should be good in studies. Do H.W, test exam preparation on her own. For math I had thought should be good but fear (as I had in childhood) of maths. Exactly same thing occurred. A day before maths exam or test she use to cry though she knew everything. She did like this only before Math. I had thought baby should score around 90% and late in higher classes around 70%. Exactly same trait has occurred.

Extra Curricular Activities: Favorite pass time – If a girl should stay at home, listen music for some time, this trait has occurred. This I kept in mind, wanted this come in baby exactly it has occurred.

Eating habits: Unlike Ist delivery I wanted baby should eat both veg and non veg. I liked my father in laws eating habit he used to relish all type of food. After eating his plate use to remain clean. Same when my daughter eats her plate at the end remain clean.(nothing left in the plate). She takes all things what ever prepared. This is to be noted that my father in law was dead during my second pregnancy. I wanted to see that does any habit or trait of dead person comes in baby if kept in mind. Yes it has occurred. I had thought should eat very little quantity should eat rice less. Should like idli. I have habit of eating tit bits in the evening. This I did not want in this baby to avoid fatness. This time I thought child should eat potatoes because is easy to cook and easily every time available (unlike my sons time). She likes to eat Potato.

Dressing up Habit: I had thought should like to have lots of clothes and fascination for clothes (like my husband) should love to dress up nicely. Exactly this trait also appeared.

Money Spending Habits: Like my husband should spend on clothes spend freely. She spends as my husband do. But at the same time I had thought should save a little. She does.

Making friends: During second pregnancy we had friction among our friend circle. Which disturbed me. So I had in mind the child should not go for friend. Should not roam after friend. As my husband do should like to stay aloof. She is exactly same. For which I am repenting. Here it shows that how environment affects.

In problematic situation: I did not think much only this much that if any hot discussion should keep mum but say only one or two sentence which would make the concerned person speechless.

Inter relationship: Should love its elder brother (my first issue), should take advice off him, should share eatables. Should be ready to sacrifice for him. My daughter is having exactly all this traits. I had thought should have coordination. Another thing I wanted she should be very much attached to me in childhood.. She happen to be same. She never leave me. Always stick type with me.

Another thing like my brother in law who liked to sit with close relatives and chat for hours, I thought and this has occurred. To see whether leader's quality comes. Yes I had thought only for very few time that like Swami Vivekanand who in his school days used to attempt all the questions and used to write on top, check any 5. She had those habit in lower classes, even having choice she used to attempt all the question. (again non generic trait)

Does quality of any actor/actress come: I had in mind Jaya Bhaduri's character in Jawani Deewani carrying doll always. My daughter carried mostly with her doll, even now she sleeps with her teddy bear.

House hold work: I had thought child should be self dependent in cooking for itself when ever hungry. She is from the age of ten self dependent in this matter. She used to prepare dosa, sandwich, omelets etc. I need not to worry if I am out of the house.

About nature: I had thought should be little arrogant like my sister in law should take decision about home affairs. Should talk less with outsiders. But love to talk with family members.

Physical features: I being on fatter side wanted my baby if girl should be like mother in law – very thin delicates but eyes like mine straight hair like mine. I thought of shape of legs like mine but fingers nicely shaped like my husband. I thought of cheeks shaped like mine. Small face like my mother in law. Jaws like my husband, neck, flat tummy like my husband. All these traits has occurred.

Study and Career related :Should study well and do job oriented course. Now she is Company Secretary and doing well.

Question arises – Is there control of pregnant women's mind over genes. Can baby be designed through mother's mind.

CHAPTER FIVE

Survey and Analysis of 120 Ladies :

This survey was done in the year 1995 – March.

I selected 120 mothers at random of different age groups, different socio economy status. Its all calculation graph has been provided. I had prepare questionnaire for survey (attached here).

Few examples : 1) Mrs. Abha's husband was not that intelligent but she herself was. She thought children to be intelligent like her, also should participate in extracurricular activity. Both traits has occurred.

2.) Washer man's wife Mrs. Chandel thought during all three pregnancies that children should be like her mother in law in nature i.e. quiet and calm minded and should study well. They were calm and took interest in study.

3.) Dr. Mrs. Nadkarni during her third pregnancy said shlokes of Sanskrit while worshipping. That child learnt and said at the age of 2.

4.) Mrs. Meena and Mrs. Usha are co sister in law lived in joint family. Mrs. Meena during her first pregnancy liked personality of elder brother in law child happens be like elder uncle. While during third pregnancy came in mind personality of husband having negative traits like alcoholic, in the child occurred that quality. Mrs. Usha during her 4[th]pregnancy kept in mind (how to avoid negative qualities).

(not purposely) like younger brother in law negative trait of alcoholism. This trait occurred in the son.

Sometimes negative traits do come in mind though pregnant woman does not like them. Sometimes due to fear some pregnant woman discuss about negative trait, to them through this counseling, that can be avoided and opposite of it can be drawn in their mind. For example the negative quality of laziness is there in her mind, we can tell her about activeness of child in work, studies and other household work.

Mrs. Chitnis thought for the first baby during pregnancy to be medico and specialist in pediatric. The daughter is doctor and a pediatrics – Question arises can mother select the career for the baby in womb.

Mrs. Mridula had liking for engineering career, this she kept in mind for whole 9 months, son Atul is IIT engineer settled in USA.

Mrs. Bhavani (Delhi) had liking and wanted baby in fetus to be IAS officer fair intelligent. Son was at the time of survey IAS officer (45 years of age) Director in Industrial Dept.. The survey also shows other features like those who kept in mind complexion features those occurred in baby.

Anita – She agreed that they both husband wife were not good looking (little ugly type). She said she purchased a sweet child's poster from the market and put on the wall. She wanted baby's face to be round, better complexion and good looking. She said she got all these traits in their son, even I saw when the child 8 years around, was exactly same.

Concerned with Studies :

Any Other :

Any idea or thinking or liking about Vocational aspect or Studies :

Do you think Child developed those qualities to which extent :   1 - 5

1	2	3	4	5
☐	☐	☐	☐	☐

Do you think what ever ocurred was

How much by chance :

How much by thinking :

Any book or photograph was concerned or was impressed by any particular person or relative :

Any - Ve habit or quality occured, which was in mind at the time of pregnancy :

Describe your Child

Quality :

Habits :

Age Now :

Rating :

Questionairre Blank

Name : *Pooja Gulati*

Age Now :   20-30   30-45   45-60   60-75

Income Group :   0-5000   5000-10,000   10,000+

Kind of family ;   Joint   Independent
During Pregnancy   [✓]   [ ]

Sr. No. of Child : *2nd*

Name of Child : *VICHAL GULATI*

Did you have awareness about thinking at the time of pregnancy ;
Grade   0   1   2   3   4   5
[ ]   [ ]   [ ]   [✓]   [ ]   [ ]

State of mind ; At the time of pregnancy.

Extremely low						Extremely high
Unhappy	1	2	3	4✓	5	Happy
Tensed	1	2✓	3	4	5	Relaxed
Excited	1	2✓	3	4	5	Calm
Free	1	2	3✓	4	5	Busy
Sick	1	2	3	4	5	Healthy

What did they think about Child at the time of pregnancy ?
wanted a healthy baby boy

About physical features ;   Nose,   Eyes,   Tall,   Complection   etc.

Nature :   Like -   Calm,   Cool,   Cheerful,   Short tempered   etc.
ofcourse little naughty and happy go lucky.

Questionairre Filled

CHAPTER SIX

SELECTED COUNSELLING AND FOLLOW UP STUDY

From 1990 I started counseling pregnant woman. I have been counseling pregnant women of all categories. Educated, uneducated even sometimes when I see pregnant woman at public places like temples, hotels, big stores etc. I must have counseled many pregnant woman. I have kept record and I do follow up study. Some of them are:

1. Mrs. Sapna – She had daughter who died (5 years). She was pregnant for third time. She wanted all the qualities like that of the daughter (dead). i.e. should be very intelligent, active cheerful. That child was good in drawing and reciting on stage. Even physical features, complexion, that child was well behaved. Mrs. Sapna had come for counseling to me. When she delivered after few months she told me she delivered a boy and that child looked exactly like previous child. It had all these traits, smiling, cheerful looks, features etc. what she percepted.

2. Dr. Preeti –She wanted baby to be like her husband. In appearance child is exactly like him. Her husband is surgeon very intelligent. Child is also very intelligent. She wanted child should do HW on its own. Child is exactly having same traits which she has thought. Even physical features height etc.

3. Mrs. Vatsala – Another close relative who was pregnant, I told her think that child should be good in studies and well behaved like herself. Where as husband who was not interested in studies and not well behaved was fair tall. I told her features complexion physique etc. like father. Should

be smiling, she percepted the same.. Exactly like what I discussed with her. It is very good is studies, score around 98% is fair always smiling. Liking to go to school. Does all HW on its own, very well behaved. Fair like father.

4. Mrs. Ashima – The young lady staying next door was pregnant and I counseled her, both are not fair but she thought of fair child, smiling, interested in studies. Should dance in marriage and parties family functions. Child was 2 years old,at the time of survey, is always smiling, dance very nicely in family functions etc. Recognizes A-Z alphabets, when mother calls for studies shows very much interest. She thought like her husband should be interested in computer related field and study in that field and build a career in computers. (Recently after 20 years again we met and the child is studying in UK in computers.)

5. Mrs. Mamta – Had come for counseling. During her pregnancy she wanted her baby in fetus – fair complexion, blue eyes (like her father) husband and herself do not have these traits like her father. When the child was born has blue eyes and fair complexion.

6. Mrs. Meeta (year 1995) – I counseled her, she herself had flat nose. I told her to think again and again of her husband's nose i.e. pointed but small. Regarding psychological traits child should have i.e. good expression, bold should communicate nicely sharp child. Now the girl is 5-6 years. She has pointed nose like father and all above mentioned traits.

7. Mrs. Ruby – I counseled her during second pregnancy. Her 1st son was my student was intelligent but shy with inhibition to talk, did not mix up with people easily. During second pregnancy I advised her (she also wanted) child should speak a lot like her father in law. Intelligent mix up with all and have good expressions, child is around two and half years. All above mentioned traits have been found.

8. Mrs. Farzain – I counseled her during 1st and 2nd pregnancy. 1st time wanted hyper active child (I told her for active) look like father, chubby cheeks, intelligent good expression dimple on chin (non genetic traits) bald (less hair) child is now 5 years. It is exactly what mother had kept in mind. Child is hyper active doesn't sit at one place, very intelligent prompt answering, good grasping power. Regarding physical features it has dimple on chin (this she wanted like her brother in law i.e. sister's husband(when born was very less hair bald from front, chubby cheeks. During her second pregnancy she wanted baby to be like elder brother (1st issue) but quiet child should sleep well at night. The baby is having

exactly same traits as thought by mother. It sleeps well at night looks like elder brother very quiet type.

9. Mrs. Sunita – She herself is fair and good looking she said husband is not that good looking. She wanted child to be like herself also like her elder son. Should be active sharp intelligent. When child was born it looked exactly like herself. Like her first son very intelligent, sharp and active.

10. Mr. Kinari – During counseling she said baby should be fair like herself but features to be like her husband i.e. big eyes, sharp nose. Unlike her husband and mother in law should mix up with every one. Baby girl when born was exactly same. Very fair complexion like mother and eyes, nose like father. Child mixes up with every one goes to everybody. is quiet and calm but intelligent.

11. Pooja said, during counseling, they both were not good ,rather less than average in studies. I told her, she also agreed that the baby in the womb should be very intelligent , interested in studies and should score well in test and exams. The son born is now 14 years old . Is very intelligent, takes interest in studies, scores more than 95 percent. As thought takes part in extra curricular activities, gets awards ,stands first or second. Pooja is very happy.

Some Typical cases

I counselled a pregnant woman Manju, It was her second pregnancy, she said my first baby daughter has problem of constipation now I want baby should get fresh every morning and easily, smoothly. I met her after 15 years , she said yes that trait has come. Same she had said when the child was 6 months old.

Two pregnant ladies when pregnant ,lost their husband. I counselled. Shweta thought for cheerful, active, intelligent. The boy is same.

Bela thought for calm and quiet type, balanced . The girl born was same.

Ashwini her self was polio patient. When she was pregnant ,I counselled, the baby girl born is now 16 years, good, understanding type, helps in all house hold work, good in studies.

It is not always that I get very favourable attitude from pregnant women. There are 4---. 5 ,because of anger on husband or any other reason ,did not pay attention, refused to take my counselling. The children born are not so good, nor taking much intrest in studies and carreer. One of them agreed, repents, for not listening. Now she herself is sending other pregnant women to me.

Other women counseling

Maid servant's daughters Seeta ,Geeta ,Lata bais daughters, Usha maids daughter in law - they all got traits in their children what they wanted after my counselling. The children were with higher IQ, took interest in studies, doing home work, preparing for exams etc.etc. One of them started counselling other pregnant woman in her neighborhood and relatives

There were two-three pregnant ladies who wanted average IQ, because they were themselves highly qualified and wanted child should not have that worry and load.

Thus there are many cases in which every lady has different opinion. Some want like father, husband, brother themselves not necessary all traits from same person. Traits can be selected from different persons, even some traits belonging to person with whom pregnant woman has no genetic relation like brother in law, sister's husband, sister-in law, co-sister in law etc. possible.

Thus we see traits of great leaders,characters from the film can be obtained.

CHAPTER SEVEN

BIOLOGICAL BASIS

The study is incomplete without the biological basis, because of the same.I tried and searched some research studies related to my work they are thus

"Latest research suggests that the foetus can hear, feel, dream, even enjoy the flavour of the curry mother eats. Behaviorally speaking there's little difference between a newborn baby and a 32 week old. It likes to be read stories, it can recognize it's mother's voice and its personality traits have already begun to develop." – By Janet L. Hopson.

Foetus learning starts in womb according to experiments and research by Fifer.

Foetus personality starts developing in womb - research and experiments of Prof. (psy.) Anthony Jame Decasper and colleagues of university of north Carolina at Green Bore, USA. Same also said according to experiments and research by Dipietro.

Very thing, all traits are carried by genes. A person's personality traits, career he opts, his life span, diseases, even suicide and divorce are in genes. There are billions of genes. <u>Genes stimulates the brainof a person</u>– result of which person shows particular behaviour pattern. Clock genes are responsible for a particular behaviour shown at particular stage of life. Like if pregnant woman thinks child should be career conscious around 15-16 years of age, that particular trait will occur that time only.

The biological basis for my study may be vice versa process. <u>That isbrain and thinking process of pregnant woman stimulates anddesigns the genes of the foetus.</u> If pregnant woman thinks baby should be intelligent or fair. The genes responsible for that trait get stimulated and occur in foetus. Few other possible biological basis are there such as autonomous nervous system of foetus, hormonal secretion of pregnant woman get effected by keeping positive traits in mind. The genetic researchers agree that there is some psychological basis for genes.

Diagram showing the correlation between genes and brain is depicted as follows:

SHAILA'S RESEARCH WORK FOR PREGNANT WOMEN

In addition to this some more bio-logical basis can be provided

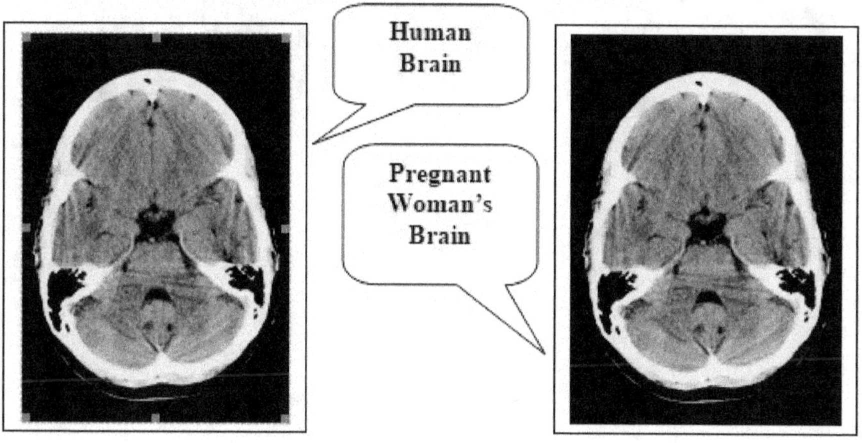

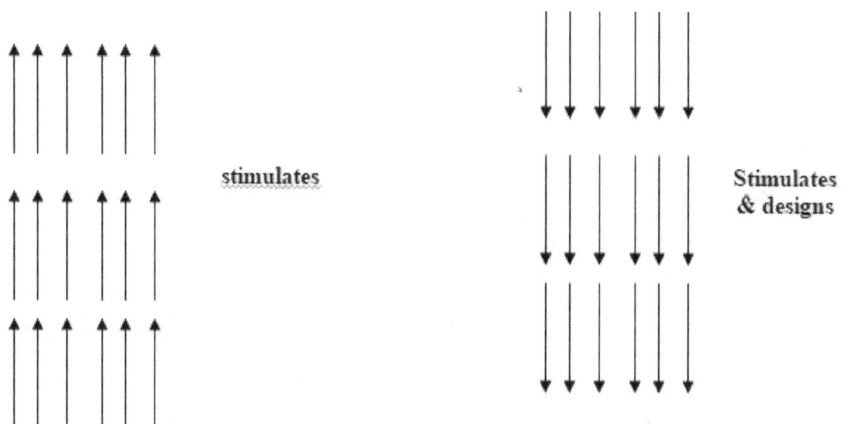

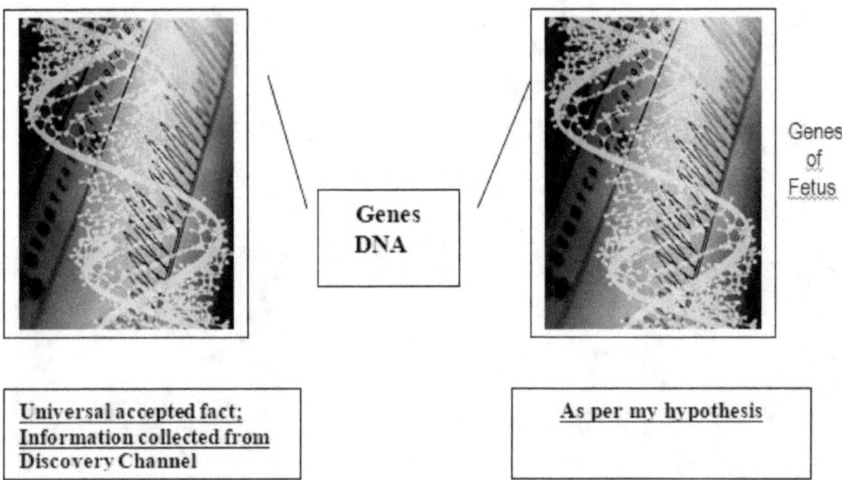

Universal accepted fact;
Information collected from
Discovery Channel

As per my hypothesis

Conclusion

Life span or age of the fetus

Now Pregnant woman can write the fate of the fetus.

Counseling other pregnant women

Nupur thought for good teeth allignment for the fetus, she got it.

Anita Chandel thought fetus to be like brother, the child is now 21 years old ,is exactly like brother. Looks wise ,height, carreer wise.

Recently I counselledNeha baby is just one month old. They are dusky in complexion wise. During counseling I told her to think for fair complexion, she agreed and the baby girl is fair..

I have counselled maid servants also. Even they could understand the phenomena nicely, rather they believed more and easily and they followed. To my great astonishment children are between 4 months to 20 years . I am getting results. Yes they get all the good qualities related to I Q level, studies,carreer, looks, caring for mother etc etc.

Till now, as I am counseling pregnant women I am getting the favourable astonishing results. Many of them come by themselves and happily tell me results.

How to remove negative traits

Pregnant woman's mind is simple tool which help her to get desired traits in fetus. Can write fate of the fetus. This tool we can control with our counseling. This counselling is a sort of remote control for her mind.

Now in this era, I would like to talk to Hon Prime minister Shri Narendra Modi's mother, if she can share her pregnancy Experiences during Modi's birth, that how this great man took birth, with such fine personality.

Can any pregnant lady produce celebrities .YES according to my theory.

I have gone through life history of many celebrities, found that during fetus stage mother had thought for such personality and that speciality. One example of singer ,director ,actor Sonu Nigam . In a TV programme he himself narrated that his mother had thought the baby in the womb should be a singer like great singer Lata Mangeshkar. And Sonu Nigam is same.Beside this I have read about many celebs, some where in their roots that speciality is there.

That speciality may or may not be in the genes or family, if pregnant woman keeps in mind, it will occur.

I wanted to do the counseling to Actress Aishwarya Rai Bacchan. So that she can produce like legend actor Amitabh Bachan.

Tennis player Sania Mirza .

Comments after counseling by pregnant women or other mothers who come with them

Sapna said oh its so nice, mam you should get Noble prize for this.

Smita said ,had come from Guahati, in this way this world will be an ideal world.

A husband who came with his pregnant wife said ,any thing else may come or not only HW doing on its own should come.

One lady who was pregnant woman 's mother in law said we have done some good deed that we met you.

One of maid servants said are you an astrologer.

4. --- 5 pregnant women said we want baby to be like you.

One gentle man said ,if I would have been in place of my pregnant wife I would have thought for a scientists and if a baby girl a painter.

Many mothers said if we could have met before, how nice it would have been. Even lady doctors said the same.

A senior citizen man had come with his daughter, said tell all pregnant women to think that child should listen to parents.

One Doctor had come with his wife, he said madam dont go on looks or IQ .The baby which comes should be an ideal person.

A woman had come from Delhi, her father in law was manufacturing and business of chemicals, said to his daughter in law, start thinking and learning names of chemicals.

Many pregnant ladies whom I had counselld long back they meet and say we can never forget you and your counseling.

Many have started giving tips to other pregnant women.

One lady whom I had counselld, she met a pregnant woman in train and gave her tips.

Even one of my maids smart daughter in law counselld her relatives and near by pregnant women.

Even I myself say 4-- 5 points to pregnant women if I met on road, in garden, airport, temples, hotels ,restaurants, malls even twice outside washroom at public place like airport, marriage hall etc etc.

Till now I have counselled pregnant women through internet, phone, book ,card,one to one counseling at home which I feel the best.

When my article was published in local news papers. At that time who were pregnant they followed and later ,after birth of child reported that they were highly benefitted. Among them one said ,my in laws side are all intelligent and fair and good looking. She said she thaught the same. And she got the same. Thus reading through news papers effected. In the same way reading through this book will also effect surely.

At the end with folded hand I Request you all pregnant women. Give birth to an angel.good human being.

Even I got excellent results with lower socio economic status. Maid servants catagory pregnant women after counseling got results that their children happily went to school, studied well by them selves, scored good marks in test ,exams.

Thus we see no economic status, iq level,only this information helps the pregnant women to get best to best results. I feel such counseling should be made compulsory for pregnant women. Also digital form should be provided to pregnant women, so that within a click it reaches to them.

Method of counseling.

After one to one personally counseling pregnant women, I tell them to come every month once at least. Second time to see what is in pregnant woman's mind I tell them to say what they want in their fetus. If any nagative thing, I tell them to correct, and tell them what is correct. They should visualise a little that how at that age level, how the baby should be. In my counselling pregnant woman has to think according to different age level.

What yet to be studied.

Can we decide span of life for fetus. Like 80 years of age with fit all the time and self dependent. Is it suggestable sudden departure from world. It is long term process. The pregnant women should write down, what traits they thought for fetus, during pregnancy only.Because I have seen in my study, some pregnant women forget what they had thought. Rather they asked me, what you had told. I give references that we had this discussion. Also many times I had remember that what they wanted.

As Biological/genetic basis ,the brain of the pregnant woman stimulates the genes, so while reading this book or during counseling on phone or personally the mind is stimulating genes of fetus .

For better effect of counseling I have prepared an album for pregnant women, it consist of nice pictures, with that a line telling of a good trait.In a picture lady has to search good features ,traits etc.Every where even in surrounding environment, she has to pick good traits. If suppose she faces some negative quality or trait ,she should immediately think opposite of it.

During counseling

I see when I tell them that baby in fetus should be smiling, a smile comes on their face, also when I tell them few other good traits like high IQ ,and caring a sweet sparkle come on their face. Which may create inner good environment producing good harmones .Thus this counselling directly or indiredtly good stimulator.

CARD

Only going through card is also helpful.

Around ten years back I gave a card to my friend Doctor, Gynaecologist requested her to get ,photo copied and distributed this card to every pregnant woman (free) . The results were overwhelming. Pregnant women liked and demanded very much. My Shaila card was in great demand.

Post Script

1)causes for suggested traits not occurring, that some ladies do not listen or to what we say.

2)Some ladies forget what.I had suggested. Rather they asked me ,you tell me what you had told me to think.

3) To pregnant women

Please to make fun.or in.anger do not think for negative traits. It will be very painful to pregnant women after the baby is born. My counselling experience has faced such.experiences.

4) Pregnant women should visualise that at.that particular stage of life what is required and should think accordingly.

5) Even circumstances surrounding effect a lot. If the circumstances are negative surroundings are negative , pregnant women should think opposite of surroundings at the time of pregnancy. For example if in surrounding situation there is laziness, she should think for activeness. If there is failure she should think for success every where.

1)Pregnant women should write which traits she wants for the baby in fetus ,at different stages of life.

After delivery she can match , at different stages of life.

Post script

A lot effects the age of the pregnant women. Young who are pregnant at the age between 20 --- 30,will think more lively things.

At the age of 30 __ 40. Will be more matured , the traits thought will be more matured type.

Also surroundings and circumstances will effect. If negative will effect to bring negative traits but pregnant women must think opposite and add positive traits.

Any thing too much is not good. Pregnant women should try to balance towards normality.

Some times pregnant women add some negativity after positive trait like

My baby should be active and not that lazy. It is wrong, should think only,

my baby should be active cheerful

Frequently Asked Questions

Ladies generally ask how can we decide traits for boy or girl. I say some traits are applicable for both like intelligence, hardworking, should be always happy, good adjustment quality etc etc. Even 1 experimented on myself second time ie if girl should be delicate and if boy should be rough and tough. It worked with me. My daughter is delicate.

FAQ

How many times should we think?

I reply it is roughly at least once in a day . My study say if pregnant woman concentrate more on a trait it occurs more. The traits paid less concentration will be less ocurring.

FAQ

Does it occur at any month, even in eighth or ninth months. Yes even thought in last two or three months they also occur. Best is for pregnant women to start making personality for the fetus, the day she comes to know that she is pregnant.

Biological basis that how it occurs in eighth month also is that fetus is in very raw state, get stimulated even in eighth ,seventh month also

Results depend a lot on pregnant woman's personality. How much she understands , how much she percepts . one who is prone to studies will opt for studies. One who is towards singing will select tha traits. Many times pregnant women dislike some traits of husband or them selves, though those traits may be good for individuals or society. I met one such pregnant woman, she herself and every body in the family were highly qualified. But she wanted baby in foetus to be average in studies and enjoy life. Should dance and do outings. The reason she gave was ,she was fed up of studies and missed all the above things because of studies. So now she wanted all those things for het baby in fetus. Thus its difficult to read or conclude about what is in pregnant woman's mind.

Another example was I counselled a beautiful young lady tall.She liked fashion nicely dressing up. Less interest in studies. I told her you are so beautiful and good looking. I said you have all qualities of a girl aspiring for beauty contest or modelling etc. I said try to have a baby like Aishwarya Rai, Miss world and top class model or actress.

She said I feel it is not so good line of my liking. She said the baby must be good looking but should study well and become a chartered accountant like my brother. Her brother was chartered accountant. Good in studies. Thus its difficult to know what is in a pregnant woman's life.

Can A Pregnant Woman Write The Fate Of Her Fetus? The Answer Is Yes. How?

The story started when I was first time on family way. My mother had come to my place for delivery. She just mentioned, when she herself was on family way, when my elder sister Was to come in this world . My mother was kept at her sister in law's place.She means my paternal aunt was married in royal family related, a very high post holder man.She (sister in law) had big bungalow luxurious life with big house servants, driver, car etc in 1945 year . Lot of gold and diamonds etc. My mother said all those things were in my mind. So my sister got all those things.

I have tried to study that what ever good events pregnant woman keeps in mind, the baby in fetus gets all those things.

So the pregnant women should think keep in mind higher financial status ,good life partner loving and caring. Good events like marriage in time. Happy life good and fit healthy life.should think of good financial status.

During my first pregnancy I had thought early promotions, high post in very young age. I myself was not sure but just to experiment I kept in mind. My son got all this.

I tried to study this with others also. I read and watched in T V about celebrities. I found those events in their lives. For example through TV programme I saw in our legend singer respected Lata Mangeshkar's 75-year-old celebration, anchor singer Sonu Nigam said his mother when Sonu Nigam was in womb had thought my baby in foetus should be like Lata Mangeshkarji a great singer and should touch the name fame .

Beside all this in Hindu mythology a famous event that in MAHABHARATA

great Arjun 's wife was pregnant and she heard by Arjuna to enter in chakravhue but she slept when he was discussed how to come out. Just imagine for a moment if She would have heard and kept in mind that how to come out. THE WHOLE MAHABHARATA would have changed.

So dear pregnant women in the same way you and your fetus ' life can change after going through this counselling.

Keep good traits, events in mind for your fetus life.

Now considering scientific basis how it may be taking place in fetus is thus. As already mentioned genes get designed in fetus, so at particular that time ,the gene responsible for that particular behaviour get designed.

Secondly may be the stars moving in the universe write that fate or those events for the baby in foetus. This I discussed with a gold madalist astrologer. He said yes this may be possible. About this all is my assumption. ie may be but what is wrong in thinking good fate for fetus. Happy smooth life.

Among some mothers I have noticed what ever they discussed some negative events ,Occurred in fetus . those negative events I don't want to discuss here because this may effect your fetus ' life .

THANK YOU

HAPPY PREGNANCY

www.ingramcontent.com/pod-product-compliance
Lightning Source LLC
Chambersburg PA
CBHW050752250726
48662CB00005B/2173